TENTH EDITION

ANYBODY'S GUIDE TO

TOTAL FITNESS

STUDENT PROFILE GUIDE

LEN KRAVITZ

Kendall Hunt
publishing company

Book Team

Chairman and Chief Executive Officer   Mark C. Falb
President and Chief Operating Officer   Chad M. Chandlee
Vice President, Higher Education   David L. Tart
Senior Managing Editor   Ray Wood
Assistant Editor   Bob Largent
Editorial Manager   Georgia Botsford
Editor   Melissa M. Tittle
Vice President, Operations   Timothy J. Beitzel
Assistant Vice President, Production Services   Christine E. O'Brien
Senior Production Editor   Mary Melloy
Permissions Editor   Caroline Kieler
Cover Designer   Mallory Blondin

Cover images © 2012, Shutterstock, Inc.

Kendall Hunt
publishing company

www.kendallhunt.com
Send all inquiries to:
4050 Westmark Drive
Dubuque, IA 52004-1840

CONTENTS

Introduction

It is not enough to read about fitness and the many positive ways it may enhance your life. The purpose of *Anybody's Guide to Total Fitness Student Profile Guide* is to facilitate your process in becoming a healthier person. This guide will help you assess your fitness level, develop reasonable goals and track your progress. An important goal of this guide is to help you stay motivated in your fitness program. Your good health is a precious commodity. Make your fitness program a priority.

Attitude Check

To better appreciate your attitude about exercise and physical activity, circle your response to the following questions.

1. Do you enjoy fitness activities? — Yes — No

2. Would you rather be a physically active person? — Yes — No

3. Do you believe exercise will improve your health? — Yes — No

4. Do you feel your involvement in fitness may improve your self-confidence and self-esteem? — Yes — No

5. Are you willing to give up time out of your busy schedule in order to improve your health? — Yes — No

6. Will you commit to your workout schedule? — Yes — No

7. Are you willing to try various exercise regimes in order to find the one that best suits you? — Yes — No

8. Are you willing to be patient in reaching your fitness goals? — Yes — No

9. Are you willing to work at overcoming any obstacles that may get in the way of your fitness progress? — Yes — No

10. Do you feel fitness is a lifelong process? — Yes — No

If you agree with most of the statements then your chances of succeeding in an exercise program are enhanced. Clarify those statements with which you disagree in order to determine if there are any barriers for you to address.

Personal Health Inventory

Describe your overall health.

Do you have chronic back pain or any other ailments? (Explain)

What are some stressors in your life?

How would you describe your eating and sleeping habits?

Are you a smoker? If so, how much do you smoke per day?

Health and Fitness Evaluation List

What personal health and fitness habits satisfy you?

What health and fitness changes would you like to make?

What short-term goals (within 10 weeks) would you like to achieve?

What long-term goals (between 4 months and one year) would you like to achieve?

Autobiography

For your instructor to get to know you better, take this opportunity to write a short autobiography. Include any information about your background, education, interests, family, hobbies, fitness, diet, and health that you would like to share.

Your Personal Fitness Contract

I want to be involved in the health and fitness movement. I want my mind, body, and spirit to realize all that life has to offer me. I am ready to take the steps to make this process a reality. I am taking a pledge and making an agreement with myself to abide by the actions below.

The short-term goals I have set for myself that I want to focus on now are:

To pursue these goals, I plan to perform the following activities on a regular basis:

I plan to begin my health and fitness program on: _____

As I reach my short-term goals, I would like to reward myself with the following:

By signing this contract I am indicating my personal commitment to reaching the goals I have established for myself:

_____   Date _____

I have recruited a helper to witness my contract:

_____   Date _____

Are You Ready to Exercise?

The Physical Activity Readiness Questionnaire (PAR-Q) can be used as a simple screening for individuals beginning low- to moderate-intensity exercise. It may be useful for referring those who need additional medical screening. It was developed by the British Columbia Ministry of Health.

Yes	No		
____	____	1.	Has your doctor ever said you have heart trouble?
____	____	2.	Do you frequently have pains in your heart and chest?
____	____	3.	Do you often feel faint or have spells of severe dizziness?
____	____	4.	Has a doctor ever said your blood pressure was too high?
____	____	5.	Has your doctor ever told you that you have a bone or joint problem such as arthritis that has been aggravated by exercise or might be made worse with exercise?
____	____	6.	Is there a good physical reason not mentioned here why you should not follow an activity program even if you wanted to?
____	____	7.	Are you over age 65 and not accustomed to vigorous exercise?

If you answered YES to one or more questions

If you have not recently done so, consult with your personal physician by telephone or in person *before* increasing your physical activity and/or taking a fitness appraisal. Tell your physician what questions you answered *yes* to on PAR-Q or present your PAR-Q copy.

If you answered NO to all questions

If you answered PAR-Q accurately, you have reasonable assurance of your present suitability for a graduated exercise program.

Estimating Your Target Zone

You can estimate your exercise heart rate with the following formula.

PERSONALIZED TARGET ZONE		
Your Estimated Maximum Heart Rate (MHR)	208 – (0.7 x Age in Years)	
Your resting heart rate		
Subtract resting heart rate from estimated MHR		
Multiply by	60%	85%
Equals		
Add resting heart rate		
Equals exercise heart rate		
	Target Zone	

10-second heart rate

Divide exercise heart rate by 6: _____ to _____

Aerobic Efficiency

Step Test

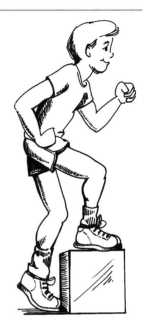

1. Select a bench, stool, or chair that is 12 inches high.

2. You will step up and down in an up, up, down, down brisk cadence.

3. Find a song that has a moderate tempo of about 96 beats per minute (16 beats in 10 seconds) to guide your cadence.

4. Rehearse stepping with the music to become familiar with the pattern.

5. Practice finding your pulse on your wrist (on the inner edge of the wrist below the base of the thumb) or at your neck (below the ear along the jaw).

6. Now, perform the stepping for three continuous minutes. On completion of the time, immediately count your pulse for 10 seconds.

STEP TEST RATING (COUNTING PULSE FOR 10 SECONDS)			
Level	**Women**	**Men**	
Excellent	16 or less	17 or less	Congratulations!
Good	17–18	18–20	Keep it up!
Fair	19–22	21–23	Begin or progress in an aerobic program
Poor	23 or more	24 or more	Start with a moderate to easy aerobic program.
(Test based on the Harvard Step Test.)			

First Test Date _____   **Retest Date** _____

Score _____   **Score** _____

Rating _____   **Rating** _____

Comments

Aerobic Efficiency

1.5-Mile Run Test

1. Establish a distance of 1.5 miles. This is six laps around most school tracks (which are usually one-quarter mile).

2. Use a stopwatch to time yourself.

3. Warm up with some easy jogging and gentle stretching before you start.

4. Cover the distance as fast as you can (running/walking). Cool down gradually at the conclusion with brisk walking for several minutes.

RATING THE 1.5-MILE RUN TIME (MINUTES)							
		Age (years)					
Fitness Category		**13–19**	**20–29**	**30–39**	**40–49**	**50–59**	**60+**
I. Very poor	(men)	>15:31*	>16:01	>16:31	>17:31	>19:01	>20:01
	(women)	>18:31	>19:01	>19:31	>20:01	>20:31	>21:01
II. Poor	(men)	12:11–15:30	14:01–16:00	14:44–16:30	15:36–17:30	17:01–19:00	19:01–20:00
	(women)	16:55–18:30	18:31–19:00	19:01–19:30	19:01–20:00	20:01–20:30	21:00–21:31
III. Fair	(men)	10:49–12:10	12:01–14:00	12:31–14:45	13:01–15:35	14:31–17:00	16:16–19:00
	(women)	14:31–16:54	15:55–18:30	16:31–19:00	17:31–19:30	19:01–20:00	19:31–20:30
IV. Good	(men)	9:41–10:48	10:46–12:00	11:01–12:30	11:31–13:00	12:31–14:30	14:00–16:15
	(women)	12:30–14:30	13:31–15:54	14:31–16:30	15:56–17:30	16:31–19:00	17:31–19:30
V. Excellent	(men)	8:37–9:40	9:45–10:45	10:00–11:00	10:30–11:30	11:00–12:30	11:15–13:59
	(women)	11:50–12:29	12:30–13:30	13:00–14:30	13:45–15:55	14:30–16:30	16:30–17:30
VI. Superior	(men)	<8:37	<9:45	<10:00	<10:30	<11:00	<11:15
	(women)	<11:50	<12:30	<13:00	<13:45	<14:30	<16:30

< Means "less than"; > means "more than."

"1.5 mile run tests," from *The Aerobics Program for Total Well Being* by Kenneth H. Cooper M.D., M.P.H, Copyright © 1982 by Kenneth H. Cooper. Used by permission of Bantam Books, a division of Bantam Doubleday Dell Publishing Group, Inc.

First Test Date _____   Retest Date _____

Score _____   Score _____

Rating _____   Rating _____

Comments

Aerobic Efficiency

Rockport Fitness Walking Test

The Rockport Walking Institute has developed a walking test to assess maximal cardiorespiratory fitness (VO_2max) for men and women. It is often helpful to do this test with a workout partner. Classes often do this test in two groups. A heart rate monitor (if available) and a watch are needed for this aerobic test.

1. Find a 1-mile course that is flat, uninterrupted, and correctly measured. A quarter-mile track is preferable for the outdoors.

2. Walk 1 mile as quickly and comfortably as possible and have your workout partner record your time at the finish mark to the closest second. For example, if a person finishes in 13 minutes and 35 seconds, the time is converted to the nearest hundredth minute by dividing the seconds (35) by 60 seconds. Thus, the time is 13.55 minutes.

3. If using a heart rate monitor, get your heart rate the instant you cross the 1-mile mark. If taking a pulse, upon crossing the finish mark immediately take a heart rate by counting your pulse for 15 seconds. Multiply that number by four to get your heart rate for one minute.

4. You can also do this test inside, especially during unpleasant weather. Walk 1 mile as fast as you can by adjusting the speed of the treadmill. Make sure you do not jog or run and keep the treadmill grade at 0% for the test. Record the time from the computer display and take your heart rate with a heart rate monitor or by taking your pulse.

5. Calculate your VO_2max using the following equation.

6. VO_2max (ml/kg/min) = 132.853 − (0.0769 × weight) − (0.3877 × age) + (6.315 × gender) − (3.2649 × time) − (0.1565 × heart rate)

   Where:

   a. Time is expressed in minutes and 100ths of a minute
   b. Weight is in pounds (lbs)
   c. Gender Male = 1 and Female = 0
   d. Heart rate is in beats/minute
   e. Age is in years

   Example VO_2max Calculations for a Female and Male:

   For a 22-year-old Female who weighs 140 lbs who completed the Rockport Walk Test in 13 minutes and 35 seconds, or 13.55 minutes, with a heart rate of 150 beats per minute the calculation would be as follows:

$$132.853 - (0.0769 \times 140) - (0.3877 \times 22) + (6.315 \times 0) - (3.2649 \times 13.55) - (0.1565 \times 150)$$
$$VO_2max \text{ (ml/kg/min)} = 45.73 \text{ ml/kg/min}$$

For a 22-year-old Male who weighs 140 lbs who completed the Rockport Walk Test in 13 minutes and 35 seconds, or 13.55 minutes, with a heart rate of 150 beats per minute the calculation would be as follows:

$$132.853 - (0.0769 \times 140) - (0.3877 \times 22) + (6.315 \times 1) - (3.2649 \times 13.55) - (0.1565 \times 150)$$
$$\text{VO}_2\text{max (ml/kg/min)} = 52.05 \text{ ml/kg/min}$$

Use the charts below to classify your cardiorespiratory fitness.

MALES: CARDIORESPIRATORY FITNESS CLASSIFICATION: VO$_2$MAX (ML/KG/MIN)						
Age	**Superior**	**Excellent**	**Very Good**	**Good**	**Fair**	**Poor**
20–30	>60	54–59	48–53	45–47	37–44	≤36
31–40	>56	50–55	45–49	39–44	34–38	≤33
41–50	>50	46–49	40–45	36–39	30–35	≤29
51–60	>46	42–45	37–41	33–36	28–32	≤27

FEMALES: CARDIORESPIRATORY FITNESS CLASSIFICATION: VO$_2$MAX (ML/KG/MIN)						
Age	**Superior**	**Excellent**	**Very Good**	**Good**	**Fair**	**Poor**
20–30	>50	46–49	42–45	36–41	32–35	≤31
31–40	>46	42–45	38–41	33–37	28–32	≤27
41–50	>41	38–40	34–37	28–33	25–27	≤24
51–60	>37	32–36	29–31	26–28	22–25	≤21

Tables derived from graphs by Shvartz, E. and Reibold, R.C. Aerobic fitness norms for males and females aged 6 to 75 years: A review. Aviation, Space, and Environmental Medicine, 61, 3–11

First Test Date	_____	**Retest Date**	_____
Score	_____	**Score**	_____
Rating	_____	**Rating**	_____

Comments

Muscular Strength and Endurance

Abdominal Strength and Endurance Test

1. Lie on your back with your hands either supporting your head or across your chest.

2. Keep your legs bent at the knees, with the feet flat on the floor about 6 to 10 inches from your buttocks.

3. To perform the "crunch," curl your trunk so that your shoulder blades come off the floor. (Your lower back stays on the floor.) Keep it smooth.

4. To take the test, count the number of "crunches" you can do for one minute.

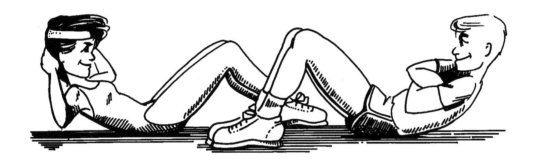

| RATING FOR ABDOMINAL STRENGTH AND ENDURANCE TEST ||
Category	Results
Excellent	60 crunches or more
Very Good	50 to 59 crunches
Good	42 to 49 crunches
Fair	34 to 41 crunches
Poor	Less than 34 crunches

First Test Date _____   **Retest Date** _____

Score _____   **Score** _____

Rating _____   **Rating** _____

Comments

Muscular Strength and Endurance

Upper Torso Strength and Endurance Test

The push-up test measures upper-body endurance, specifically in the chest (pectoralis muscles), shoulder (anterior deltoids) and arms (triceps). Due to common variations in upper body strength, women should be assessed doing the modified push-up. Men should be assessed using the standard push-up. However, as the illustration shows, for training women should do either the standard or modified push-up depending on which provides the optimal challenge.

1. The start position is with the chest lowered so it almost makes contact with the floor. Extend the arms on the upward phase.

2. To take the test, count the total number of push-ups completed in one minute.

PUSH-UP TEST NORMS FOR MODIFIED PUSH-UP (WOMEN)					
AGE	Excellent	Good	Average	Poor	Very Poor
20–29	>48	34–48	17–33	6–16	<6
30–39	>39	25–39	12–24	4–11	<4
40–49	>34	20–34	8–19	3–7	<3
50–59	>29	15–29	6–14	2–5	<2

PUSH-UP TEST NORMS (MEN)					
AGE	Excellent	Good	Average	Poor	Very Poor
20–29	>54	45–54	35–44	20–34	<20
30–39	>44	35–44	24–34	15–23	<15
40–49	>39	30–39	20–29	12–19	<12
50–59	>34	25–34	15–24	8–14	<8
Norms for men and women adapted from Pollock, M.L. et al. *Health and Fitness Through Physical Activity*, New York: John Wiley & Sons.					

First Test Date _____   **Retest Date** _____

Push-up Style _____   **Push-up Style** _____

Score _____   **Score** _____

Rating _____   **Rating** _____

Comments

Flexibility

Sit-and-Reach Test

Flexibility is specific. This means that the degree of flexibility in one joint will not necessarily be the same in other joints of the body. Because a lack of flexibility in the lower back, back of the legs, and hips is a contributing cause for 80 percent of lower-back problems of our population, this flexibility test was chosen.

1. Sit with your legs extended in front of you. Keep your feet perpendicular to the floor. Place a ruler along your legs on the floor.

2. Slowly stretch forward, reaching toward (or past) your toes and hold. (Do not bounce!) Keep your legs straight but not locked.

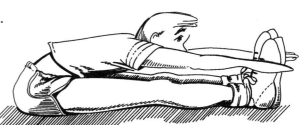

3. It is best to do this several times for practice, gently stretching further toward your point of limitation.

RATINGS FOR THE SIT-AND-REACH TEST	
Category	**Results**
Excellent	7 inches or more past the toes
Very Good	4 to 7 inches past the toes
Good	1 to 4 inches past the toes
Fair	2 inches from in front of the toes to 1 inch past
Poor	More than 2 inches in front of the toes

A limitation of this sit-and-reach test is that it does not differentiate between a person with short arms and/or legs and someone with long arms and/or short legs. However, this test is very appropriate to monitor flexibility changes over time.

First Test Date _____   **Retest Date** _____

Score _____   **Score** _____

Rating _____   **Rating** _____

Comments

Body Composition

Pinch Test for Body Fat

The pinch test is a quick check for body composition. (You can always count on the mirror to tell you a lot, too!)

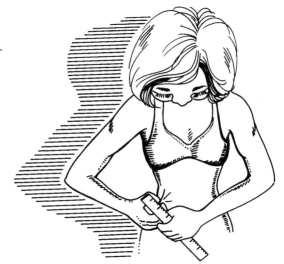

1. With your thumb and forefinger, pinch the skin and fat at the waist just above the hips. (Be sure not to pinch any muscle. Pull the skinfold away from your body.)

2. With a ruler measure the width of the pinch.

RATINGS FOR PINCH TEST		
Level	**Men**	**Women**
Good to Excellent	1/2 inch or less	1 inch or less
Fair to Good	1 inch to 1/2 inch	1 1/2 inch to 1 inch
Poor	Over 1 inch	Over 1 1/2 inch
Refer to Skinfold Caliper Measurement for a more accurate estimate of body composition.		

First Test Date _____   **Retest Date** _____

Score _____   **Score** _____

Rating _____   **Rating** _____

Comments

Body Composition

Anatomical Skinfold Sites

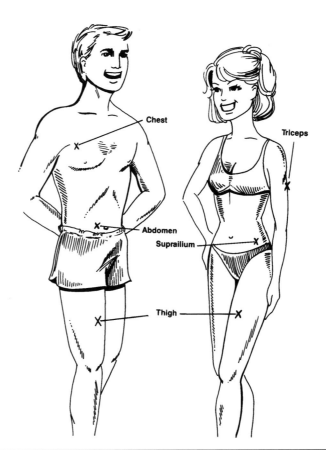

	First Test Date _____		Retest Date _____
	Score _____		Score _____
	Rating _____		Rating _____

Measurements

	First Test	Retest
Chest	_____	_____
Triceps	_____	_____
Abdomen	_____	_____
Suprailium	_____	_____
Thigh	_____	_____

Comments

Body Composition

Skinfold Nomogram

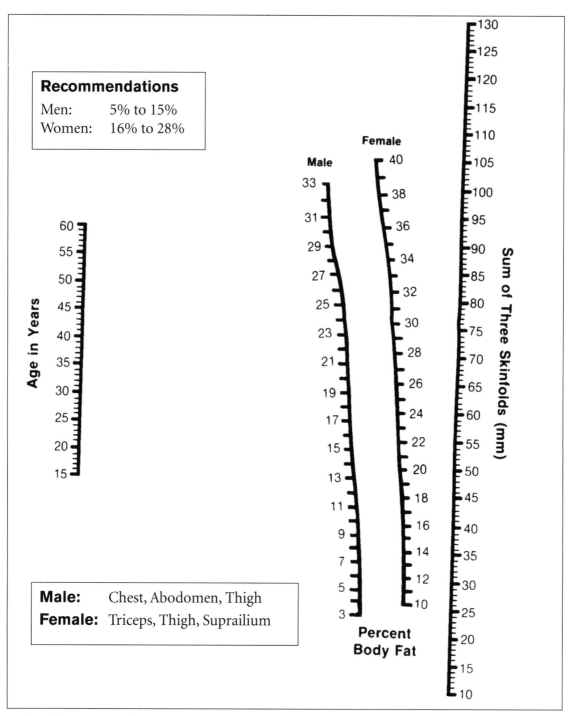

Recommendations

Men: 5% to 15%
Women: 16% to 28%

Male: Chest, Abodomen, Thigh
Female: Triceps, Thigh, Suprailium

Reprinted by permission from Baun, W. B. Baun, M. R. A Nomogram for the Estimate of Percent Body Fat from Generalized Equations. *Research Quarterly for Exercise and Sport,* 52 (1981), 380–384.

Body Composition

Target Body Weight

You can estimate your desired body weight by using your percentage of body fat. Follow the example below.

1. Your weight in lbs. ⎯⎯⎯⎯⎯⎯ 150 ⎯⎯⎯⎯⎯⎯ lbs.

2. Skinfold body fat measurement result (Round off to whole number) ⎯⎯⎯⎯⎯⎯ 22 ⎯⎯⎯⎯⎯⎯ %

3. Fat weight (your weight × item 2) ⎯⎯⎯ 150 × .22 = 33 ⎯⎯⎯ lbs.

4. Lean body weight (your weight – item 3) ⎯⎯⎯ 150 – 33 = 117 ⎯⎯⎯ lbs.

5. Desired percent body fat ⎯⎯⎯⎯⎯⎯ 17 ⎯⎯⎯⎯⎯⎯ %

6. Desired weight (item 4 ÷ (1.00 – item 5)) ⎯⎯ 117 ÷ (1 – .17) = 141 ⎯⎯ lbs.

7. Pounds to gain or lose (your weight – item 6) ⎯⎯⎯ 150 – 141 = 9 ⎯⎯⎯ lbs.

Now Estimate Your Desired Body Weight

1. Your weight in lbs. ⎯⎯⎯⎯⎯⎯⎯⎯⎯⎯⎯⎯ lbs.

2. Skinfold body fat measurement result (Round off to whole number) ⎯⎯⎯⎯⎯⎯⎯⎯⎯⎯⎯⎯ %

3. Fat weight (your weight × item 2) ⎯⎯⎯⎯⎯⎯⎯⎯⎯⎯⎯⎯ lbs.

4. Lean body weight (your weight – item 3) ⎯⎯⎯⎯⎯⎯⎯⎯⎯⎯⎯⎯ lbs.

5. Desired percent body fat ⎯⎯⎯⎯⎯⎯⎯⎯⎯⎯⎯⎯ %

6. Desired weight (item 4 ÷ (1.00 – item 5)) ⎯⎯⎯⎯⎯⎯⎯⎯⎯⎯⎯⎯ lbs.

7. Pounds to gain or lose (your weight – item 6) ⎯⎯⎯⎯⎯⎯⎯⎯⎯⎯⎯⎯ lbs.

Body Composition

Waist-to-Hip Ratio

The distribution of body fat in the abdomen, chest and lower back increases the risk for heart disease, stroke, type 2 diabetes and some forms of cancer. This regional body fat distribution is referred to as android obesity. Fat that gathers in the hips, buttocks, and thighs, called gynoid obesity, is of lower risk than the android pattern. Ideally, your hips should be larger than your waist. You can assess this risk following the steps below.

1. Use a flexible tape measure.

2. Take measurements while standing, keeping the tape measure parallel to the floor.

3. Measure the circumference of your waist at the level of your navel.

4. Measure the circumference of your hips at the greatest protrusion of your buttocks.

5. Divide your waist measurement by your hip measurement.

   Waist/Hip = _____

6. Interpretation

   Males: If your waist-to-hip ratio is 0.94 or greater, you are at a higher than normal risk.

   Females: If your waist-to-hip ratio is 0.82 or greater, you have a higher than normal risk.

First Test Date _____   **Retest Date** _____

Score _____   **Score** _____

Rating _____   **Rating** _____

Comments

Estimate Your Resting Metabolic Rate

Your resting metabolic rate (RMR) is the energy requirements the body uses to keep all your systems functioning at rest. It is best estimated with the Miflin-St Jeor RMR equations for men and women. There is no scale or ranking for RMR, it is just a useful measure of resting energy expenditure.

Males: RMR = $10 \times$ (wt in kg) + $6.25 \times$ (ht in cm) – $5 \times$ (age in years) + 5

Females: RMR = $10 \times$ (wt in kg) + $6.25 \times$ (ht in cm) – $5 \times$ (age in years) – 161

To determine body weight in kg from lbs simply divide weight in lbs by 2.205. For instance, a 140 lb woman would calculate body weight in kg as follows: 140 lbs/2.205 = 63.5 kg. Height in centimeters is easily determined by multiplying a person's height (in inches) by 2.54. So, for a female who is 5 feet 6 inches (or 66 inches), height in centimeters is 66 inches $\times$ 2.54 = 167.64 cm. So a female whose is 30 years old, 140 lbs and 5 feet 6 inches would estimate her RMR as follows:

$$RMR = 10(63.5) + 6.25(167.64) - 5(30) - 161$$

$$= 635 + 1048 - 150 - 161$$

$$= 1372 \text{ calories per day}$$

Now it's your turn to estimate your resting metabolic rate.

What is your weight in lbs?_____

Divide your weight in lbs by 2.205 to determine your weight in kg. _____

What is your height in inches? _____

Multiple your height by 2.54 to determine your height in centimeters. _____

Now choose the equation and estimate your personal resting metabolic rate.

Males: RMR = $10 \times$ (wt in kg) + $6.25 \times$ (ht in cm) – $5 \times$ (age in years) + 5

Females: RMR = $10 \times$ (wt in kg) + $6.25 \times$ (ht in cm) – $5 \times$ (age in years) – 161

First Test Date _____

Your resting metabolic rate is _____ **calories per day.**

Retest Date _____

Your resting metabolic rate is _____ **calories per day.**

Caloric Expenditure Chart

You can easily estimate the number of calories you expend during aerobic exercise activities. To determine the number of calories expended, multiply the total number of minutes of activity times the calories per minute. For example, a 110-pound woman doing 20 minutes of continuous aerobic dance would expend approximately 172 Calories (8.6 × 20 = 172).

CALORIC EXPENDITURE CHART FOR SELECTED AEROBIC ACTIVITIES	
(Aerobic dance, cycling, brisk walking, rope skipping, rowing on a machine, running, skating, and swimming.)	
Your weight in pounds	**Calories Expended per minute**
95–104	8
105–114	8.6
115–124	9.0
125–134	9.7
135–144	10.3
145–154	11
155–164	11.5
165–174	12
175–184	12.7
185–194	13.3
195–204	13.7
205–214	14.2
215–224	14.7
225–234	15.2
235–244	15.7
245–254	16.2
255–264	16.7
265–274	17.2
275–284	17.7
Values may vary from individual to individual.	

Total number of minutes of aerobic exercise   _____

Calories expended per minute according to your weight   _____

Your estimated caloric expenditure   _____

Estimating Your Caloric Needs

You can estimate the breakdown of your daily intake of carbohydrates, proteins and fats. Follow the steps below.

To estimate your daily caloric needs, first multiply your weight by 16 (if you are moderately active) or 12 (if you are relatively sedentary).

1 gram of carbohydrate	= 4 calories
1 gram of protein	= 4 calories
1 gram of fat	= 9 calories

Daily nutritional needs

Carbohydrates	= 58% of your daily calories
Proteins	= 12% of your daily calories
Fats	= 30% of your daily calories

Weight (lbs): _____ × 16 or 12 = _____ (Estimate of daily caloric needs)

Carbohydrates

Carbohydrate Calories per Day

Estimate of calories per day: _____ × 0.58 (58%) = _____ calories/day

Carbohydrate Grams per Day

Divide the above product by 4: _____ ÷ 4 = _____ grams/day

Proteins

Protein Calories per Day

Estimate of calories per day: _____ × 0.12 (12%) = _____ calories/day

Protein Grams per Day

Divide the above product by 4: _____ ÷ 4 = _____ grams/day

Fats

Fat Calories per Day

Estimate of calories per day: _____ × 0.30 (30%) = _____ calories/day

Fat Grams per Day

Divide the above product by 9: _____ ÷ 9 = _____ grams/day

PHYSICAL ACTIVITY LOG				
Date	Activity	Duration	Heart Rate or RPE	Comments

PHYSICAL ACTIVITY LOG				
Date	Activity	Duration	Heart Rate or RPE	Comments

PHYSICAL ACTIVITY LOG				
Date	Activity	Duration	Heart Rate or RPE	Comments

PHYSICAL ACTIVITY LOG				
Date	**Activity**	**Duration**	**Heart Rate or RPE**	**Comments**

PHYSICAL ACTIVITY LOG				
Date	**Activity**	**Duration**	**Heart Rate or RPE**	**Comments**

PHYSICAL ACTIVITY LOG				
Date	Activity	Duration	Heart Rate or RPE	Comments

PHYSICAL ACTIVITY LOG				
Date	Activity	Duration	Heart Rate or RPE	Comments

DAILY FOOD DIARY					
(Record all meals and snacks) Date _____					
Food	**Calories**	**Protein**	**Carbs**	**Fat**	**Sodium**
Totals					

Did you work out today? If yes, what was your estimated caloric expenditure from this workout? (See Caloric Expenditure Chart)

Total calories consumed _____

Minus calories expended in exercise _____

Equals net daily caloric consumption _____

DAILY FOOD DIARY					
(Record all meals and snacks) Date _____					
Food	**Calories**	**Protein**	**Carbs**	**Fat**	**Sodium**
Totals					

Did you work out today? If yes, what was your estimated caloric expenditure from this workout? (See Caloric Expenditure Chart)

Total calories consumed _____

Minus calories expended in exercise _____

Equals net daily caloric consumption _____

DAILY FOOD DIARY					
(Record all meals and snacks) Date _____					
Food	**Calories**	**Protein**	**Carbs**	**Fat**	**Sodium**
Totals					

Did you work out today? If yes, what was your estimated caloric expenditure from this workout? (See Caloric Expenditure Chart)

Total calories consumed _____

Minus calories expended in exercise _____

Equals net daily caloric consumption _____

DAILY FOOD DIARY					
(Record all meals and snacks) Date _____					
Food	**Calories**	**Protein**	**Carbs**	**Fat**	**Sodium**
Totals					

Did you work out today? If yes, what was your estimated caloric expenditure from this workout? (See Caloric Expenditure Chart)

Total calories consumed   _____

Minus calories expended in exercise   _____

Equals net daily caloric consumption   _____

DAILY FOOD DIARY					
(Record all meals and snacks) Date _____					
Food	**Calories**	**Protein**	**Carbs**	**Fat**	**Sodium**
Totals					

Did you work out today? If yes, what was your estimated caloric expenditure from this workout? (See Caloric Expenditure Chart)

Total calories consumed   _____

Minus calories expended in exercise   _____

Equals net daily caloric consumption   _____

DAILY FOOD DIARY					
(Record all meals and snacks) Date _____					
Food	**Calories**	**Protein**	**Carbs**	**Fat**	**Sodium**
Totals					

Did you work out today? If yes, what was your estimated caloric expenditure from this workout? (See Caloric Expenditure Chart)

Total calories consumed _____

Minus calories expended in exercise _____

Equals net daily caloric consumption _____

DAILY FOOD DIARY					
(Record all meals and snacks) Date _____					
Food	**Calories**	**Protein**	**Carbs**	**Fat**	**Sodium**
Totals					

Did you work out today? If yes, what was your estimated caloric expenditure from this workout? (See Caloric Expenditure Chart)

Total calories consumed   _____

Minus calories expended in exercise   _____

Equals net daily caloric consumption   _____

DAILY FOOD DIARY					
(Record all meals and snacks) Date _____					
Food	**Calories**	**Protein**	**Carbs**	**Fat**	**Sodium**
Totals					

Did you work out today? If yes, what was your estimated caloric expenditure from this workout? (See Caloric Expenditure Chart)

Total calories consumed   _____

Minus calories expended in exercise   _____

Equals net daily caloric consumption   _____

Notes

Notes

Notes